MESOTHELIOMA

THE KILLER

DR AUDREY WASH

Copyright©2022 Audrey Wash

All Rights Reserved

MESOTHELIOMA 1
THE KILLER 1
DR AUDREY WASH 1
Copyright©2022 Audrey Wash 2
All Rights Reserved 2
   INTRODUCTION 6
What is Mesothelioma? 6
   CHAPTER ONE 8
What Is Mesothelioma Malignant growth? 8
   CHAPTER TWO 12
Peritoneal Mesothelioma Side effects 12
   CHAPTER THREE 16
Testicular Mesothelioma Side effects 16
   CHAPTER FOUR 18
How Can You Say whether You Have Mesothelioma?...18
   CHAPTER FIVE 22
Side effects of Mesothelioma by Stage 22
   CHAPTER SIX 26
How Might I Adapt to Mesothelioma Side effects?.......26
   CHAPTER SEVEN 28

Overseeing Mesothelioma Side effects 28
   CHAPTER EIGHT 32
Individuals Most In danger of Creating Mesothelioma .32
   CHAPTER NINE 34
Phases of Mesothelioma 34
   CHAPTER TEN 36
Mesothelioma Future and Forecast 36
   CHAPTER ELEVEN 38
Mesothelioma Treatment Choices 38
     CONCLUSION 41

INTRODUCTION

What is Mesothelioma?

Mesothelioma is a harmful growth that is brought about by breathing in asbestos filaments and structures in the coating of the lungs, midsection, or heart.

Side effects can include windedness and chest torment.

The lifespan for most mesothelioma patients is around a year after analysis.

Therapy might further develop visualization and can incorporate a medical procedure, chemotherapy, or radiation

CHAPTER ONE

What Is Mesothelioma Malignant growth?

Mesothelioma is a disease brought about by asbestos openness. Mesothelioma malignant growth happens for the most part in the covering of the lungs. In any case, the disease likewise happens in the covering of mid-region and testicles.

Chance of mesothelioma malignant growth increments with delayed asbestos openness. Mesothelioma might be forestalled by staying away from asbestos.

Mesothelioma Side effects

Side effects of mesothelioma seem when cancers spread, develop and press against the chest divider and the stomach depression. Early determination can help patients' possibilities profiting from greater treatment choices. Since side effects are like those of different circumstances, an underlying misdiagnosis is normal. It's vital to know about your set of experiences of asbestos openness and examine it with your primary care physician straightaway.

Pleural (Mesothelioma of the Lungs) Side effects

- Chest torment
- Windedness
- Dry hack
- Weakness
- Dryness
- Trouble gulping
- Diminished chest development (trouble relaxing)

- Unexplained weight reduction
- Fever
- Muscle shortcoming
- Expanding of the face and arms

Whenever side effects are recognized and treated rapidly, patients might profit from a more excellent of life and a better future. Side effect control is a fundamental part of exhaustive treatment for mesothelioma in the lungs.

CHAPTER TWO

Peritoneal Mesothelioma Side effects

Early indications of peritoneal mesothelioma can be confused with stomach related conditions like bad tempered gut disorder or feminine issues like fibroids. Normal side effects of peritoneal mesothelioma, which structures on the delicate tissue covering the midsection, include:

- Stomach torment
- Stomach enlarging
- Stomach liquid development (ascites)
- Unexplained weight reduction
- Sickness and regurgitating
- Blockage
- Loss of hunger

Specialists can recommend chemotherapy drugs, for example, pemetrexed, cisplatin, carboplatin and gemcitabine, to contract peritoneal mesothelioma cancers and slow disease development.

Experts are currently seeing unprecedented outcomes with hyperthermic intraperitoneal chemotherapy (HIPEC). With magnificent side effect control and the best medicines, many individuals live longer than mesothelioma measurements foresee.

Pericardial Mesothelioma Side effects

Early indications of pericardial mesothelioma can be confused with coronary illness. Normal side effects of pericardial mesothelioma include:

- Trouble breathing (dyspnea)
- Chest torment
- Windedness
- Heart palpitations or unpredictable heartbeat (arrhythmia)
- Heart mumbles

Pericardial mesothelioma creates in the coating around the heart called the pericardium. It is probably the most uncommon type of the sickness. Side effects originate from thickening of the pericardium, which can make it harder for the heart to function well.

CHAPTER THREE

Testicular Mesothelioma Side effects

Early indications of testicular mesothelioma can be confused with injury or ailments, for example, epididymitis, which includes aggravation of the balls. Normal side effects of testicular mesothelioma include:

- Hydrocele (liquid in the scrotum)
- Testicular agony
- Enlarged testicles
- Irregularity in scrotum

An irregularity in the testicles is the most widely recognized indication of testicular mesothelioma - the most extraordinary of a wide range of mesothelioma. It represents under 1% of all mesothelioma cases.

First Indications of Mesothelioma

The earliest indications of mesothelioma threat can incorporate a hack, windedness and chest, shoulder or stomach torment. Over and over again mesothelioma isn't analyzed until side effects become extreme and patients are as of now in the later phases of this intriguing and genuine type of disease.

Knowing the principal cautioning signs and side effects, and knowing your set of experiences of asbestos openness, can assist with affirming an early mesothelioma finding. An early finding can assist you with fitting the bill for life-expanding treatments that might be inaccessible to patients in later phases of mesothelioma.

CHAPTER FOUR

How Can You Say whether You Have Mesothelioma?

A biopsy will affirm assuming you have mesothelioma. Be that as it may, specialists may initially see the early indications of mesothelioma coincidentally. A normal test, for example, a X-beam or blood tests, may identify something uncommon. Since side effects look like less genuine illnesses, they are bad marks of the disease.

Notwithstanding a biopsy, mesothelioma testing normally incorporates X-beams, CT outputs and blood tests. Specialists are chipping away at other creative tests to affirm a mesothelioma conclusion, including a breath test.

How Do Mesothelioma Side effects Add to Conclusion?

Mesothelioma side effects are the main thrust that carries patients to the specialist to start the symptomatic interaction. Since mesothelioma side effects most regularly create in stage 3 or stage 4, most patients don't go to the specialist until the malignant growth has advanced to a late stage.

Illuminate your essential consideration specialist about any set of experiences of asbestos openness. Inquire as to whether they suggest any disease screenings in view of your openness history and individual wellbeing history. Getting disease early gives a superior possibility meeting all requirements for forceful malignant growth medicines that might further develop endurance.

Since it doesn't ordinarily deliver such signs until some other time in the sickness interaction, it is hard to analyze mesothelioma in stage 1 or 2 in view of side effects alone. In any case, in certain occasions, beginning phase mesothelioma can create sufficient pleural liquid around the lung to cause windedness or hack without having spread.

A recent report found that stage 1 and stage 2 pleural mesothelioma patients who got less forceful medical procedure joined with chemotherapy, radiation treatment or both experienced the longest after finding. The middle endurance of this gathering was 35 months, or almost three years.

Mesothelioma cell type, epithelial versus sarcomatoid, doesn't change the run of the mill side effects experienced by most patients with this malignant growth.

CHAPTER FIVE

Side effects of Mesothelioma by Stage

A mesothelioma patient will encounter side effects that contrast from stage 1 to arrange 4 mesothelioma. The size of cancers and how far they have spread decides the stage order and the area and size of growths straightforwardly impacts the patient's side effects.

Beginning phase MESOTHELIOMA Side effects: STAGE 1 AND STAGE 2

- Dry hack or wheezing
- Windedness
- Trouble relaxing
- Torment in chest or midsection
- Pleural radiation (liquid development), prompting demolishing torment and breathing challenges

LATE-STAGE MESOTHELIOMA Side effects: STAGE 3 AND STAGE 4

- Expanded and more determined torment
- Iron deficiency and related weariness
- Weight reduction
- Loss of craving
- Respiratory intricacies
- Trouble gulping
- Entrail Impediment

Factors That Effect Mesothelioma Side effects

Little cancer size is the fundamental explanation mesothelioma patients don't encounter side effects in the beginning phases of the disease's development.

Mesothelioma growths normally don't turn out to be large to the point of affecting the body until late phases of disease improvement including stage 3 and stage 4.

•   Chest Torment: Essentially because of cancers spreading into the chest divider and its nerves.

•   Trouble Relaxing: Brought about by cancers confining full extension of the lungs.

•   Pleural Radiation: Results from growths spreading widely into the pleural coating or lymph hubs in the chest. This keeps liquid from appropriately depleting out of the pleural hole, which confines the lung from growing.

As cancers develop, they start to put strain against and develop into neighboring organs and tissues. As penetrating malignant growth tissue pack and compromise tissues and organs, they start to glitch, and, in the end, this prompts organ disappointment.

CHAPTER SIX

How Might I Adapt to Mesothelioma Side effects?

Numerous malignant growth habitats presently offer palliative disease care that might incorporate physician recommended drug, exercise based recuperation, word related treatment and different methodologies that work on your everyday existence and keep your side effects in charge.

Mesothelioma side effects result from the malignant growth itself and might be like a portion of the symptoms of disease treatment.

Results of disease treatment as a rule reduce days to weeks after treatment closes. Mesothelioma side effects will generally advance as the disease propels. Side effect the board is basic to personal satisfaction.

Converse with your oncologist about a reference to a palliative consideration subject matter expert. These specialists work in side effect the executives and keeping up with or working on personal satisfaction.

CHAPTER SEVEN

Overseeing Mesothelioma Side effects

•   Elective Treatments: Strong integral and elective medicines, for example, needle therapy and brain body treatments, are displayed to assist patients with overseeing torment, tension and sickness.

•   PleurX Catheter: This permits the patient to deplete the liquid at home each 2-3 days with the assistance of a little silicone catheter.

•   Radiation Treatment: Radiation treatment alone won't fix mesothelioma, however it can recoil growths and alleviate agony and strain.

•   Correspondence: Let your PCP know about changes in type or power of your side effects. This will permit your PCP to suggest different systems or treatments that will fundamentally diminish distress and torment.

- Mesothelioma Subject matter experts: Mesothelioma is an interesting sickness and looking for care from a mesothelioma specialty specialist can work on your admittance to state of the art treatments demonstrated to further develop side effects and draw out endurance after conclusion. Treatment plans might remember investment for clinical preliminaries or remedies for immunotherapy prescriptions. While progress rates for immunotherapy treatment change for every understanding, these drugs have shown guarantee and the U.S. Food and Medication Organization has endorsed Keytruda, Opdivo and Yervoy for harmful mesothelioma treatment.

Tracking down a Trained professional

Assuming you have a background marked by openness to asbestos and accept your side effects show mesothelioma, look for sure fire clinical consideration. Enlighten your PCP regarding past work around asbestos and alarm them to the chance of an asbestos-related sickness. Request a second assessment from a mesothelioma subject matter expert if necessary.

CHAPTER EIGHT

Individuals Most In danger of Creating Mesothelioma

Individuals most in danger of creating mesothelioma malignant growth dealt with asbestos for a drawn out timeframe or were presented to a lot of word related asbestos. Handed down openness is additionally normal, particularly among the life partners and offspring of individuals who worked with asbestos. Veterans were likewise uncovered while serving in the U.S. military.

- Veterans
- Firemen
- Technicians
- Chimney stack clears
- Diggers

- Development laborers
- Air conditioning experts
- Material plant laborers
- Circuit testers
- Relatives

CHAPTER NINE

Phases of Mesothelioma

Organizing tracks threatening mesothelioma cancer development and assists specialists with making a therapy arrangement and anticipate patient guess. The phases of mesothelioma range from 1 to 4 and depend on growth size and area.

Beginning phase mesothelioma is more bound to one site, while late-stage mesothelioma shows growths spreading past the chest or stomach hole. Arranging is a significant piece of deciding treatment.

- Stage 1

The disease is confined. Medical procedure is best at this stage. Endurance rate is higher. A patient's middle future at stage 1 is 22.2 months.

- Stage 2

Cancers have spread from the first area into contiguous constructions. Medical procedure is as yet a choice. The life expectancy for each patient at stage 2 is 20 months.

- Stage 3

Malignant growth has spread into territorial lymph hubs. Medical procedure is a choice in select cases. The life expectancy for each patient at stage 3 is 17.9 months.

- Stage 4

Growths have spread into far off organs. Chemotherapy and immunotherapy ease side effects. The life expectancy for each patient at stage 4 is 14.9 months.

CHAPTER TEN

Mesothelioma Future and Forecast

At the point when specialists examine a mesothelioma disease patient's anticipation, they are deciding the general standpoint for that particular person. Commonly, when patients ask about their mesothelioma guess, what they're keen on is data about future.

While there is no fix, the viewpoint for every tolerant changes relying upon elements, for example, the patient's age, generally wellbeing, how early a determination is made and assuming their forecast can be improved with treatment and the reception of a solid way of life.

Key Variables

Stage and cell type are factors that most influence mesothelioma guess. Age, orientation and by and large wellbeing additionally influence viewpoint. More people have a preferred mesothelioma guess over more established men. Individuals determined to have the peritoneal mesothelioma type likewise have a more prominent possibility of endurance.

Ways Of further developing Guess

Eating a supplement rich eating routine, remaining sound, going through disease medicines and settling on a better way of life decisions can further develop harmful mesothelioma visualization and prosperity. For instance, stopping smoking and getting influenza and pneumonia immunizations further develops lung capacity and by and large wellbeing.

CHAPTER ELEVEN

Mesothelioma Treatment Choices

Mesothelioma disease is treated with customary treatments like a medical procedure, chemotherapy and radiation, as indicated by the most recent review in the American Culture of Clinical Oncology. Arising malignant growth medicines, including immunotherapy, are additionally accessible for certain patients. However few out of every odd patient is qualified for each sort of mesothelioma disease treatment, most patients can profit from palliative consideration to assist with overseeing side effects.

- Medical procedure

These techniques are utilized for diagnosing sickness, eliminating cancers and facilitating torment. Extrapleural pneumonectomy or pleurectomy and decortication medical procedures offer the best opportunity of endurance for patients with solid wellbeing and restricted malignant growth spread.

- Chemotherapy

Over 70% of patients go through chemotherapy. The treatment's solid medications contract growths and kill disease cells yet in addition accompany treatment aftereffects.

- Radiation Treatment

Radiation treatment can be controlled at any disease stage. Specialists use it to diminish torment and slow cancer development. It is regularly joined with a medical procedure and chemotherapy.

- Immunotherapy

Immunotherapy drugs control disease development and assist some mesothelioma patients with living longer. Specialists use immunotherapy at any stage, and achievement rates fluctuate for every persistent.

- Cancer Treating Fields (TTFields)

This FDA-endorsed disease treatment treats pleural mesothelioma. TTFields works in mix with chemotherapy to restrict disease development and further develop endurance.

- Clinical Preliminaries

Scientists and specialists offer these exploratory treatments to qualified patients the country over. Mesothelioma clinical preliminaries can prompt new or further developed medicines.

CONCLUSION

Most specialists have never experienced mesothelioma since it is an uncommon disease. Specialists who center around mesothelioma at specialty treatment focuses give patients the best possibilities broadening life and further developing anticipation.

A review distributed in the Diary of General Inward Medication affirmed that disease care requires "abilities of specialty doctors like clinical oncologists, specialists and radiation oncologists."

Printed in Great Britain
by Amazon

24729030R00030